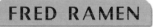
FRED RAMEN

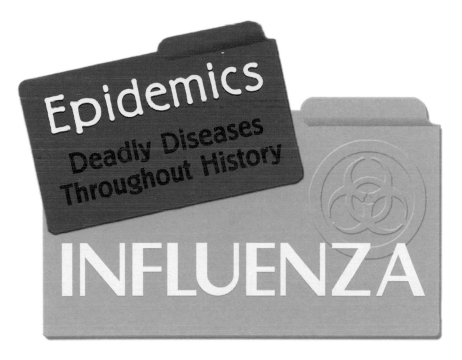
Epidemics
Deadly Diseases
Throughout History

INFLUENZA

The Rosen Publishing Group, Inc.
New York

For Jeff Mackin

Published in 2001 by The Rosen Publishing Group, Inc.
29 East 21st Street, New York, NY 10010

First Edition

Library of Congress Cataloging-in-Publication Data

Ramen, Fred
Influenza / by Fred Ramen. — 1st ed.
    p. cm. — (Epidemics)
Includes bibliographical references and index.
    ISBN 0-8239-3347-4 (lib. bdg.)
    1. Influenza—History—Juvenile literature. [1. Influenza.
2. Epidemics. 3. Diseases.] I. Title. II. Series.
    RC150.4 .R36 2000
614.5′18′09—dc21
                                        00-009380

Cover image: An electron micrograph of the influenza A virus.

Manufactured in the United States of America

CONTENTS

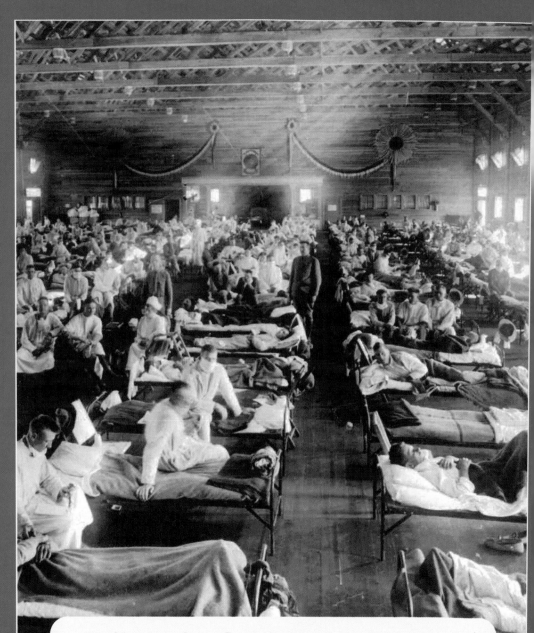

In this 1918 photo, flu victims crowd into an emergency hospital at Camp Funston in Kansas.

INTRODUCTION

World War I—which pitted Britain, France, Russia, and their allies against Germany, Austria-Hungary, Turkey, and their allies—was raging. It had been four years of bloody fighting in which millions of soldiers lost their lives. They had been slaughtered by machine-guns, choked to death by deadly gases, or blown to bits by long-range artillery. And millions of civilians were impoverished and suffering from hunger—especially in Germany—because most nations' money and resources were going to support the military. But no advances were being made on either front. The war maintained a steady state of stalemate.

Then, in the spring of 1918, the German army launched an ambitious plan to break out of their trenches, smash through northern France, and capture Paris, the heart of the country. It was a desperate plan, made more desperate by the fact that the entire country of Germany was near collapse. The British had successfully blockaded goods going into the country, slowly starving German civilians to death. But the Germans had one advantage: They had recently signed the Treaty of Brest-Litovsk with the newly formed Soviet Union. The treaty ended the fighting on Germany's eastern front. The Germans were now able to use the soldiers who had been fighting the Russians to fight the French and British.

For the first few weeks, the German plan succeeded brilliantly. The Allies—Britain, France, and those countries that were fighting with them—were driven back. Many French troops became so demoralized by being beaten so badly in various battles that in several instances they refused to continue attacking the Germans. In danger of losing the war once and for all, the French and British commanders begged their new ally, the United States (which had entered the war only at the end of the previous year), to send more troops as fast as possible. The United States granted its allies' request. But in doing so, a new horror was set in motion, one that eventually not only stopped the German army dead in its tracks and brought it stumbling toward certain defeat, but would eventually kill more people than the war itself. Many of the American troops who landed in Europe that year were sick with a new strain of influenza, the Spanish flu, a strain that would in time prove to be perhaps the deadliest plague in human history.

Disease and warfare have gone hand-in-hand throughout human history. In fact, until the second half of the twentieth century, a soldier was far more likely to be killed by disease than by an enemy soldier. Whenever armies were on the march, plague was sure to follow. And this was never more true than during World War I. It created the perfect environment for a terrifying epidemic.

1

THE SPANISH FLU

In March of 1918, American soldiers training in Camp Funston, Kansas, suddenly came down with a particularly strong strain of the flu. Many of those who got sick contracted pneumonia because their bodies were so weak from having been so ill. All told, forty-eight soldiers died from the flu-induced pneumonia. This flu, while unusually infectious, received little notice; the deaths from pneumonia were unfortunate but not uncommon for the time.

Not long after the flu outbreak in Kansas, flu outbreaks were reported in Europe, where American troops were being rushed to help fight against the massive German attack. Soon, soldiers on both sides were infected with the flu. Massive epidemics were reported all across

Europe. This early strain of the flu, however, was not yet as deadly as it would become and actually seemed to be fading away by the end of summer.

In August of that year, however, new cases of the flu began to be reported in army camps. At Camp Devens, outside Boston, over 17,000 soldiers developed the flu between August and October, and 727 of them died. Although many had died from other ailments like pneumonia, streptococcus (strep), or staphylococcus (staph) infections, many others had died from nothing more than the flu itself. This indicated to doctors that they were dealing with a very strong strain of influenza.

The symptoms of this flu were especially severe. The soldiers would, in addition to the normal flu symptoms, develop nosebleeds. They would often cough up blood or bloody mucus. Their skin would turn blue. Soon after exhibiting these symptoms, they would die. Autopsies found that their lungs were filled with a bloody froth. The flu was causing fluid to pour into their lungs, rupturing the tiny air sacs called alveoli where oxygen enters the bloodstream.

This was the Spanish flu, so-named because initially more cases were reported in Spain than in the other European nations. This was to be the twentieth century's greatest pandemic. (A pandemic is a disease

ca. 3000–2000 BC
Influenza first becomes capable of infecting humans. Probably arises in central Asia.

412 BC
Hippocrates describes influenza.

AD 1387, 1580, 1610
Possible dates of first European epidemics.

1500s
Spanish soldiers, who destroyed the Aztec Empire of Mexico, spread a new strain of influenza that caused several epidemics.

outbreak that spreads over a wide area and affects a large part of the population.) The Spanish flu killed at least 20 million people worldwide between 1918 and 1919, although many authorities believe the actual number was higher. Some estimate the number of deaths at 30 or 40 million people.

Ripe for Infection

The world was ripe for an airborne infectious disease in 1918. The war was bringing together people from all over the world and confining them in unsanitary trenches and camps. Indians in the

1833
First worldwide pandemic of influenza.

1890–91
Russian flu sweeps through the world; deadliest influenza pandemic in history at that point.

1918
March: First strain of Spanish flu emerges in the United States.
September: Second wave of Spanish flu breaks out in the eastern United States and Europe.
October: Second wave peaks. Thousands die in cities across the world.

(continued)

British army fought beside Senegalese from Africa and Americans from New York City. People's immune systems were no doubt already taxed by the sudden exposure to unfamiliar diseases. Now, crammed together for long periods of time, the soldiers were perfect targets for contracting influenza. Soon the armies of both sides were heavily stricken by the new, deadlier infection. The German attack, already slowed by the presence of fresh American troops in the battlefield, came apart as fewer and fewer soldiers were available for duty. Soon the Germans were in retreat, with the Austro-Hungarian Empire teetering on the edge of collapse.

1919

Third wave peaks. New York is hit hardest at this time. In Paris, U.S. president Woodrow Wilson, attending the peace talks that have ended World War I, contracts the Spanish flu. Although he survives, some historians cite his illness, which left him substantially weakened, as the reason he unexpectedly gives in to the French demands for a harsh peace with Germany.

1920

Spanish flu disappears from humans. Pigs in the midwestern area of the United States begin to contract a new type of swine flu.

1933

Scientists successfully isolate the influenza virus.

An epidemic that had been confined to the soldiers of the armies would have been bad enough. But influenza soon spread to the civilian population. Soldiers trained in camps near the cities and many would return to those cities when they were on leave. When the war ended in November of 1918, many more rushed back to their homes. They made those journeys home on ships and in railway cars crammed with people. This was the perfect environment for infecting large groups of people in a short time. In America, the cities of the East Coast were infected by the early fall.

1957
Emergence of a new influenza strain starts the Asian flu pandemic.

1976
A new kind of influenza emerges in pigs that causes severe infections in humans. Quick production of a vaccine, however, prevents a world-wide pandemic.

1999
A new kind of influenza strain, which can infect humans directly from birds, emerges in Hong Kong.

1968
The Hong Kong flu, a new strain of influenza, starts another worldwide pandemic.

The Flu Comes to America

The hardest hit East Coast city was Philadelphia. In late September of 1918, the city began to post warnings about the flu. Within two weeks, the city was overwhelmed by influenza. Almost immediately, the city began to feel the strain of dealing with the new, deadly infection.

A major obstacle to combating the disease was the war effort. America was in a patriotic fervor in 1918. The resources of the entire nation were being turned toward fighting the war in Europe. Patriotic rallies were held for thousands of people, bringing them all

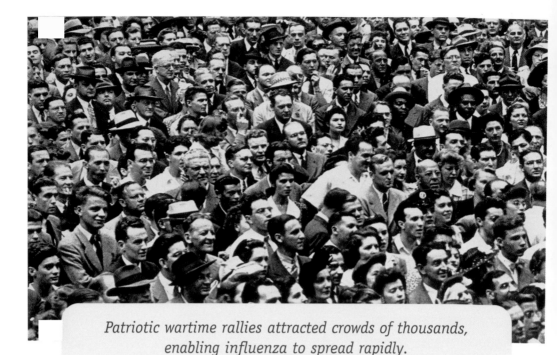
*Patriotic wartime rallies attracted crowds of thousands,
enabling influenza to spread rapidly.*

together in small spaces—perfect arenas in which
they could be exposed to the deadly influenza virus.

Public health officials did what they could to prevent the spread of influenza, but their own lack of
knowledge as to its true cause and the need to focus
most of their efforts on helping overseas troops hin-
dered them. On September 28, Philadelphia held a
war bond rally that attracted thousands; just five
days later, with flu spreading like wildfire, the city
closed all schools, saloons, churches, and theaters.

While well-intentioned, the order did little to stop
the spread of influenza. As long as people rode poorly
ventilated streetcars and elevators, and worked in
stuffy office buildings, the disease would spread.

By the week of October 5, over 700 people had died in Philadelphia from the flu and pneumonia. Over 7,000 would die in the next two weeks. Many thousands more were bedridden by the disease. The city's institutions began to break down quickly. Policemen, firemen, and sanitation workers were often too sick to work. Hospitals were swamped with victims for whom very little could be done. Soon, doctors and nurses were becoming sick as well. Nurses were especially in demand; even today, there is little that doctors can do for someone who suffers from influenza other than try to alleviate the symptoms. For this reason, nurses were far more important than doctors. In most cases, all a person needed to recover from the flu was bed rest, fluids, and someone to help with his or her basic needs. During the worst part of the epidemic in Philadelphia,

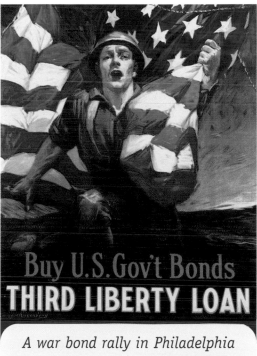

Buy U.S. Gov't Bonds
THIRD LIBERTY LOAN

A war bond rally in Philadelphia caused the flu to spread throughout the city in just five days.

the city was accepting anyone, trained or not, who could care for the sick.

There was still another crisis in the city: the unburied dead. Nothing could break a population's morale during an epidemic more than the sight of unburied corpses piled up throughout the city. Also, the corpses were unsanitary and a breeding ground for other diseases. The city used the existing war supply committees to solve the problem: Businesses that had woodworking equipment were asked to produce coffins, and by the end of the epidemic, over 2,000 coffins of various types had been made. Prisoners and volunteers from throughout the city dug graves to bury the dead. Steam shovels were used to dig ditch graves for those too poor to buy individual plots. By the middle of October, as the disease began to retreat, the unburied dead were no longer a problem.

Although Philadelphia was strained almost to the breaking point, somehow the city and its people found ways to cope. Not only was every doctor and nurse in the city mobilized for flu duty, but medical students and nurse trainees were forced to deal with situations they would not normally have encountered for years. To avoid straining them further, a special phone number, "Filbert 100," was set up and staffed twenty-four hours a day. People could call the number for doctors, ambulances, or other assistance. Strain was further reduced by sending people to the houses of flu sufferers for a "preliminary visit." Often, those who were suffering needed only advice and encouragement. These house visits cut the number of hospital visits by about a third.

All of the city's organizations—religious, social, political—joined in the effort to combat the flu. Catholic nuns nursed the sick. The Patrolman's Benevolent Association (the policemen's union) supplied off-duty policemen to act as stretcherbearers. Business owners in South Philadelphia voluntarily closed down their shops and distributed food and medical supplies. The Automobile Club volunteered cars to serve as ambulances. Many people volunteered their services, knowing that they were putting themselves in the path of a deadly disease. In the end, while the war effort did much to spread the disease, the spirit of volunteerism that the war inspired did much to help Philadelphia combat the flu.

The flu, which had first struck in earnest during the first week of October, began to subside during the last week of the month. On October 27, churches were reopened; the next day, schools reopened, and all bans were lifted by October 30. Less than a thousand people died of the flu or pneumonia in November; by the end of that month, the epidemic was over. From the end of September to the beginning of November, nearly 12,000 people had died of the flu and its related infections; many others probably died of unrelated causes, such as heart trouble, that became deadly to their flu-weakened bodies. Philadelphia had passed through a great crisis, and survived. Its one good fortune was that it had to deal with one wave of infection. Others cities, such as San Francisco, had to deal with several waves.

Influenza Continues Its Rampage

San Francisco had one major advantage over the East Coast cities: a warning that influenza was coming. By the end of September, the public health officials of the city were already considering what steps they needed to take to contain the flu. They were sobered by the example of Seattle, where 10,000 people came down with influenza after attending a review of the National Guard Infantry, an event that brought several thousand people together. But even though this information was known, several massive rallies were still held in San Francisco at the end of September and the beginning of October.

Soon influenza exploded throughout San Francisco. By October 14, almost 1,000 cases had been reported; by the end of the next week, the schools, churches, and theaters had all been closed, and there were 4,000 new cases of the flu.

As in Philadelphia, many of the city's basic services broke down. Garbage piled up along the streets because the garbagemen were too sick to make their rounds. Firemen and policemen were also often unavailable. The telephone service nearly stopped working when too many of its operators fell ill.

The flu hit San Francisco's poor and immigrant populations hard, especially those living in the city's famous Chinatown. Crammed into crowded dwellings, often distrustful of the authorities and frequently ignored by them, San Francisco's Chinese population suffered greatly during the epidemic.

Dr. William Hassler, chief of the city's board of health, launched an aggressive and ambitious campaign against the disease. Besides the usual methods of closing public facilities and calling out all medical personnel, including dentists and medical students, Hassler tried two other techniques: vaccines and masks.

Vaccines—which, at that time, were made to fight the bacteria commonly found in flu victims—had also been attempted in Philadelphia toward the end of that city's epidemic. They were totally ineffective, but since they were introduced toward the end of the flu's rampage, people believed that the vaccines might have helped. Vaccines were introduced in San Francisco at the start of November, which was near the end of the first wave of infection in that city. This once again fooled many into believing that it was the reason why the epidemic subsided.

Masks were a more controversial plan. The idea was that masks of gauze, like the ones surgeons wear today, would somehow filter the influenza germs out of the air. Today we know this is impossible; the influenza virus is far too small to be filtered by gauze. But because no one knew this at the time, the city, at Dr. Hassler's urging, passed a mask ordinance, or law, that required anybody who was out in public to wear a mask.

Although the ordinance did not take effect until November 1, San Franciscans, haunted by the fear of death, rushed to get masks. By October 26, more than 100,000 masks had been distributed throughout the city. The number of new flu cases dropped by over 1,000 in the week following; a week later, the number of new cases dropped by nearly 5,000. By the middle of November, the epidemic seemed to be over.

Although the campaign seemed to have been a success, and Hassler was congratulated for stopping a major epidemic, there had been problems all along with the masking law. Many people found them

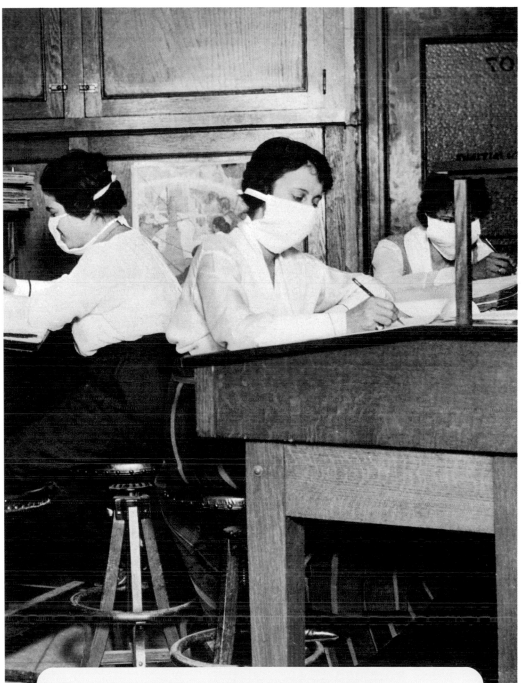

An ordinance was passed in San Francisco
that required people to wear masks.

extremely uncomfortable to wear; others felt they were not proper for a democratic society. People often removed them to smoke, or followed the letter of the law by leaving them tied to their faces but hanging below their chins. Even though the number of flu cases had dropped dramatically in November, Hassler refused to do away with the ordinance while he felt that there was still a danger of infection. It wasn't until November 21 that the citizens of San Francisco were legally allowed to remove their masks.

Just over a week later, however, the number of new flu cases began to increase again. By the middle of December, it was clear that a second epidemic was in full bloom. Although the horror of late October, when 1,300 people had died in two weeks, was not repeated, the second wave would kill over 1,000 people in the month of January alone. Hassler immediately put the mask law back in place, against much public resistance (including an attempt to plant a time bomb in his office). The people were forced to begin wearing masks again on January 17. And again there was an immediate drop in the number of new cases. On February 1, the city was once again able to unmask. Over 3,500 people had died in the two flu waves. Although it seemed like the precautions of masking and vaccines had worked, neither had really had any effect. One example of how ineffective the masks were was that over three-quarters of the nurses, who wore their masks all the time, fell ill. It would be decades before any really effective defense against influenza would be devised.

2

INFLUENZA THROUGHOUT HISTORY

Influenza is probably as old as human civilization. It is difficult to know exactly when humans first began to catch the disease. This is not only because there are few records that survive from the beginning of human history, but also because the symptoms of influenza are not very different from colds and other more common and less deadly infections. Also, influenza normally kills only the very young and very old—people who, for most of human history, were already in the greatest danger of dying from disease, making it difficult to tell precisely what killed them.

The reason we believe influenza to be as old as human civilization is because many domesticated animals, such as horses, pigs, and chickens, also can catch forms of the influenza virus. In fact, the most common way for a new strain to spread to humans is for them to catch it from their pigs. Because of this, scientists believe the disease probably originated in wild animals that were domesticated by humans. Eventually, a form of the disease arose that could be caught by humans, who were spending enough time with their animals for diseases to be spread between them.

The common symptoms of influenza are those of a severe cold. However, the onset of symptoms is usually much more rapid. Within a day or two of being infected, the disease makes its presence felt. The infected person suffers from a high fever, chills, and muscleaches (this last symptom is the best way to tell if you have the flu or just a cold). The respiratory tract—the nose and throat—become inflamed and raw; sneezing, coughing, sore throat, and a runny nose all result. The infected person usually feels very weak and unable to get out of bed. Within three or four days, the symptoms subside, although people who have caught the disease may not recover their full strength for weeks or even months.

Influenza rarely kills healthy people. Infants and young children, whose immune systems (the body's natural defense against disease) are not yet fully developed, and elderly people, whose immune systems have weakened with age, can be killed by it. Influenza kills either by causing the lungs to fill with fluid, literally drowning the infected person in his or her own body, or by weakening the immune system and allowing other diseases such as pneumonia and bronchitis to invade the body.

Epidemics!

It is difficult to say when the first flu epidemics began. Hippocrates, a Greek physician known as the Father of Medicine, described the disease in 412 BC. Medical researchers have combed through old records and give various dates—1387, 1580, 1610—for the first epidemics in Europe. The influenza virus has a characteristic that makes it both very successful at infecting people and difficult to track: It tends to mutate, or change, very rapidly. This means that people are more likely to be exposed to a strain they have never encountered before, and thus have no resistance to; it also means that the virus tends to disappear after about a year because the strain has mutated so much that it is no longer infectious.

In previous centuries, when people rarely traveled far from home, it was difficult for influenza to become a true pandemic since the strain would usually die out before it could be transmitted to enough

Influenza may have been spread by the
Spanish conquerors of the Aztec Empire of Mexico.

people over a wide enough area. But as Europeans began to explore the world, using faster and faster methods of travel, the virus began to spread just as fast. There is evidence that the Spanish soldiers who destroyed the Aztec Empire of Mexico in the 1500s spread not only the deadly smallpox virus to the Americas, but a new strain of influenza, which caused several epidemics. And Europe experienced several epidemics during the eighteenth century that spread across the continent. But the first worldwide pandemic, which spread as far as the Far East and the Americas, took place in 1833. The 1833 virus was especially virulent, or infectious; it infected half the population of Europe and killed tens of thousands.

The First Modern Pandemic

The first pandemic of the modern age was that of 1889–90. It seems to have started in central Russia, the apparent point of origin for most of the European epidemics of the eighteenth and nineteenth centuries. For the first time in history, there was a rapid system of transportation, in the form of steam-powered trains and ships. This dramatically contributed to the spread of the disease throughout the world. Numerous populations were infected before the virus could mutate to a less deadly form. For the first time, Europe and the Americas were infected at the same time with the same flu virus, thanks to the speed and volume of transatlantic shipping. The disease also spread at nearly the same time into Asia and Africa. Over 250,000 people died in Europe alone, a far greater number than from the more feared diseases, cholera and smallpox.

Yet despite the numerous deaths and great amount of sickness, the pandemic was quickly forgotten. The flu, the silent killer, was ignored in favor of other, less common diseases. But ignoring this disease has had tragic consequences.

The Spanish Flu: Smaller Outbreaks

Trying to forget the Spanish flu, and not thoroughly researching it, was a mistake from which people

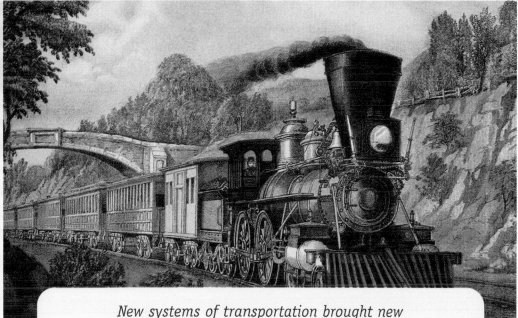

New systems of transportation brought new ways of spreading disease with them.

continue to suffer. Not only did the disease affect the countries involved in the war, it spread to all parts of the globe during its several months of existence. In Alaska, where the population was isolated by severe winter weather, attempts to block the flu by means of quarantine helped only a small amount. As many as 2,000 of the territory's Native American population died from the flu, showing no resistance to it at all. In faraway Samoa, only a strictly enforced quarantine put in place by the U.S. Navy and aided by the islanders themselves prevented disaster; the British-controlled regions of Samoa did not put such measures in place, and 8,500 people— 22 percent of the population—died. The Spanish flu killed thousands of men on board the transport ships that carried them between America and Europe. Again, the cramped conditions of the ships were ideal for the spread of the flu. And almost 18,000 people died in Paris of influenza or pneumonia.

And then suddenly it was gone. By 1920, the disease had vanished as mysteriously as it had come, apparently leaving no traces. Perhaps as many as 40 million people had died throughout the world. Yet, curiously enough, the Spanish flu seemed to fade from people's memories as soon as it stopped infecting people. After five years of war and disease, people seemed to want to be unburdened of their troubles; the Roaring Twenties, the Jazz Age, began. The Spanish flu was forgotten.

The Spanish flu was a medical disaster. Doctors could do nothing to stop its spread. The measures they did take were totally ineffective. They could find neither the disease's cause nor its cure. Yet people seemed to forget or overlook this as well. They continued to believe that medicine would one day conquer all infectious disease. But as history has shown us, it would take well over half a century for that illusion to be shattered.

3

HUNT FOR THE KILLER

A medical revolution had taken place in the hundred years before the Spanish flu. The causes of infectious diseases, so long a mystery to human understanding, had finally been discovered. Scientists knew diseases were caused by microscopic organisms that attack the body's cells. Even at the time of this discovery, methods such as the smallpox vaccine had already been developed to fight infectious disease. Thanks to the work of such pioneers as Louis Pasteur and Robert Koch, many disease-causing bacteria and viruses had been isolated and vaccines had been created that prevented people from becoming infected. By the beginning of the twentieth century, it seemed that the long battle with infectious diseases would soon be won.

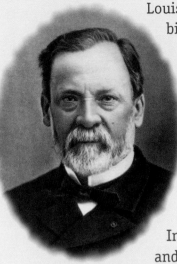

Louis Pasteur

Louis Pasteur (1822–1895), a French biologist, was one of the most outstanding scientists of the nineteenth century. His work caused our understanding of disease to take a giant leap forward.

Pasteur is best known for his work in microbiology. In the 1850s, he studied fermentation and demonstrated that it was caused by microscopic organisms. In the 1860s, he developed processes and techniques that could inhibit the growth of these organisms. Named after the scientist, pasteurization techniques allowed the transportation of milk and other spoilable goods over a much greater distance than before.

But Louis Pasteur's most outstanding work came in the area of vaccination. Pasteur was able to isolate the organisms responsible for many diseases, such as anthrax (a disease of sheep and occasionally humans), chicken cholera, and a disease of silkworms that threatened to destroy the entire French silk industry. In the 1880s, he was able to perfect techniques of producing a weakened rabies virus that could be used to create a vaccine for the disease, which until then had been incurable.

Pasteur's virtues were those of an ideal scientist: He constantly experimented and attempted to reproduce and verify his results. His outstanding successes brought a new level of scientific precision to biology.

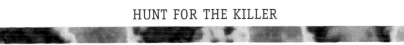

Yet the best scientific minds of the early twentieth century were unable to understand the Spanish flu. They could not cure it, stop it from spreading, create a vaccine for it, or even isolate its cause. In the years that followed the horror of the influenza pandemic, many scientists attempted to find out exactly what had caused the Spanish flu, and how to create an effective flu vaccine. The hunt for the killer was on.

The Search for a Cause

One problem the scientists encountered was a complete misunderstanding about what caused influenza. Although scientists knew about viruses, they didn't really understand them. And in 1918, no one believed influenza was caused by a virus. They believed it was caused by a kind of bacteria known as Pfeiffer's bacillus.

Richard Friedrich Johann Pfeiffer was a German bacteriologist of considerable skill who studied influenza after the great pandemic of 1890–91. He discovered bacteria growing in great quantities in the upper respiratory tracts of people with the flu. This bacteria was named *Haemophilus influenzae* in the belief that it caused the flu, but it was more commonly called Pfeiffer's bacillus.

Although Pfeiffer believed he had found the cause of influenza, there were some problems with his research. Although he was able to infect monkeys and rabbits (the latter, it is now known, are not able to catch influenza) and produce flulike symptoms, autopsies showed that the tissue did not have the same damage as that caused by influenza, nor was he able to find the bacteria in large quantities every time. He was thus unable to fulfill the last two of Koch's postulates (see page 36) and could not definitely prove that Pfeiffer's bacillus caused the flu.

Nevertheless, Pfeiffer's enormous reputation as one of the nineteenth century's best bacteriologists caused many scientists to ignore their doubts and believe that the bacteria caused the Spanish flu.

Richard Friedrich Johann Pfeiffer and Robert Koch

The fact that it was often found in the lungs of patients who died from the flu seemed to support this belief. However, many people who died of the flu had other infections, such as staphylococcus or strepto-coccus infections. And still others had apparently died of no obvious bacterial infection.

Another problem that scientists faced in their hunt for the cause of influenza was that humans were the only animals known to contract it. Humans, obviously, make bad laboratory animals. It is difficult to control human behavior in such a way as to limit contamination by other diseases. And obviously it is not ethical to infect humans with deadly diseases. Until a laboratory animal could be found that contracted influenza and was able to then pass the disease back to a human, research would have to depend on analysis of people who had caught the disease, making it extremely difficult to isolate and study.

A third frustration was that the mechanisms of how a virus works were not yet fully understood. To grow, or culture, a bacteria, one merely needs to find something that the bacteria likes to "eat" and then place a sample of the bacteria into that sub-stance. Viruses, on the other hand, need to invade a living cell in order to reproduce; they cannot be cultured in the same way as bacteria. Nowadays, it

Robert Koch (1843–1910), a contemporary of Louis Pasteur, further refined the techniques of identifying the causes of infectious disease. An outstanding laboratory technician, Koch perfected the method known as "pure culture," in which a certain type of bacteria was grown without contamination from any other bacteria. This made it possible to test for which bacteria caused the disease.

At about this time, Koch formulated his four postulates for determining which microorganism is the cause of a particular disease.

1. The microorganism must be found in every case of the disease, existing in a relationship with the damaged tissue of the patient in a way that explains that damage.

2. The microorganism must be grown in a pure culture outside the patient.

3. This culture must be able to produce in healthy animals an illness that is identical in all respects to the original disease.

4. The microorganism must then be recovered from the infected animals.

Koch himself is best known for discovering the life cycle of the anthrax bacteria, the bacteria that causes tuberculosis, and the bacteria that causes cholera. His work furthered the scientific revolution in medicine begun by Pasteur.

is easy for scientists to use eggs or cells taken from a living organism to culture a virus, but these techniques were far beyond the understanding of the early flu researchers.

Gradually, however, scientists began to chip away at the secrets of the origin of the flu. Various tests conducted throughout the 1920s demonstrated that the cause of influenza was not a bacteria, although some still held that it was caused by a poison secreted by a bacteria. Meanwhile, research on a different disease, found only in animals, finally provided the techniques and knowledge needed to isolate the flu virus.

Canine distemper is a disease of dogs. Although humans cannot catch it, the symptoms are very similar to those of the flu. In the early twentieth century in England, the disease killed many of the dogs used in foxhunting. In 1926, the virus that causes distemper was isolated, and a vaccine was in production by 1929. Scientists had also developed a number of techniques, such as separating the research animals from the outside world and sterilizing all equipment brought into the research area, that would prove to be valuable in flu research.

They had also discovered an ideal laboratory animal: the ferret, which was even more susceptible to distemper than dogs. In 1933, during a flu epidemic in England, a group of scientists, theorizing that the flu

Influenza is caused by a virus. A virus is a small, but very dangerous organism. It is not alive in the way that you or an animal or even bacteria are alive. It cannot reproduce on its own. In order for a virus to make more viruses, it must invade the cell of a living being. Because viruses are very small, no one even figured out that they existed until the middle of the nineteenth century. And it wasn't until the twentieth century that special microscopes called electron microscopes allowed humans to see and take photos of them.

A virus is made up of proteins—one of the essential building blocks of any cell—and a substance called RNA. RNA is essentially a set of instructions for how to build a cell, or in this case, a virus. Normally, a cell will use RNA to maintain the health of the part of the body for which it is responsible. When a virus enters a cell, however, it substitutes its RNA for the cell's. Instead of working to maintain the body's health, the cell now makes more viruses. These new viruses then invade other cells and turn them into virus factories. This is how the infection spreads. "Influenza" comes from the Italian word for "influence." It was believed that the influence of bad stars was causing the disease. Influenza infects the cells of the respiratory tract—the organs in your body responsible for breathing—and causes a person to sneeze. When he or she does, thousands of viruses are spread in the droplets of water expelled by the sneeze.

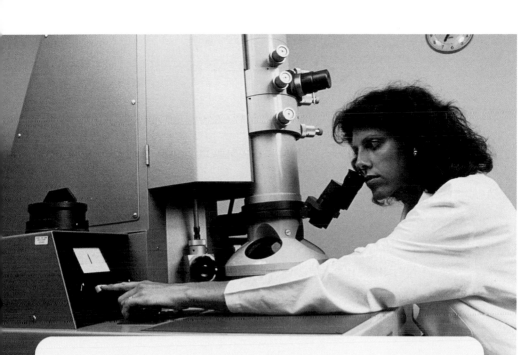

Electron microscopes allow researchers to see and study viruses.

was caused by a virus, decided to use ferrets as test subjects. Using infected matter taken from humans suffering from influenza, they managed to infect several ferrets with a disease that resembled influenza. They were then able to infect healthy ferrets using material taken from the sick ferrets. Tests on the blood samples of humans who had recovered from the 1933 flu showed that they had developed antibodies to the virus taken from the ferrets. And in 1936, a sick ferret sneezed in the face of a scientist, who soon developed symptoms that were undoubtedly those of the flu. The virus had at last been discovered.

At about the same time scientists discovered another crucial piece of the puzzle: the swine flu. The swine flu is a type of influenza that infects pigs and is the same as human influenza. In fact, swine flu outbreaks in the United States after 1918 were caused by the remnants of the Spanish flu virus. It was quickly proven that horses and many domesticated animals also catch influenza. Currently, scientists believe that influenza first arises in birds. The strain mutates and eventually becomes able to infect pigs and horses, who then pass the disease on to humans.

THE FLU TODAY

The Spanish flu, although the most deadly flu outbreak, was not the last influenza pandemic of the twentieth century. Since 1918, there have been two other pandemics, the 1957 Asian flu and the 1968 Hong Kong flu that together killed more than 1.5 million people. And in 1976, a new strain arose in pigs that caused severe illness in human beings, but rapid production of a vaccine prevented a pandemic.

The rapidly changing nature of influenza continually produces new strains. Several different strains are now currently infecting humans around the world. However, the great danger is the emergence of a new strain that humans have never before encountered. Such a strain would have the high infection rates that

41

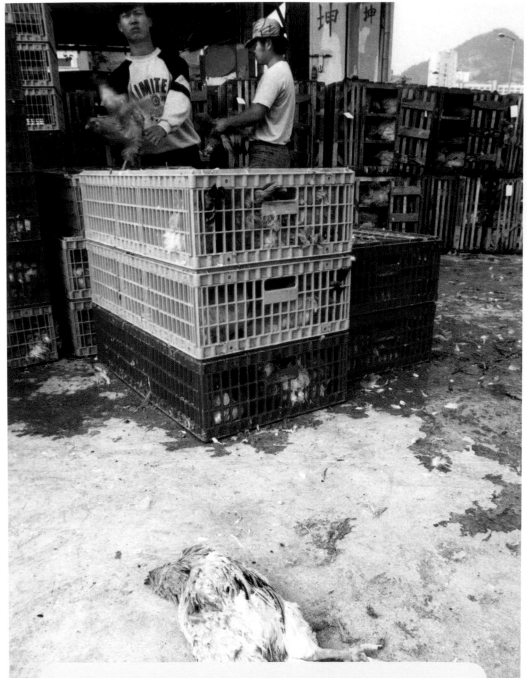

Thousands of chickens were slaughtered in Hong Kong in an attempt to control an influenza outbreak.

diseases always have when introduced to new populations; the fear is that it might be as lethal as the Spanish flu.

In 1999, several flu cases in Hong Kong were found to be caused by a new strain of influenza. This strain was unique because it had been transmitted to humans directly from chickens, rather than pigs or other mammals. Influenza that could be transmitted to humans directly from birds could be much more dangerous than other strains, as birds have a much greater range of influenza strains and can travel farther than most mammals. The outbreak was contained in Hong Kong by slaughtering thousands of chickens, but international health organizations continue to monitor the growth of this new strain.

Dangers of Rapid Mutation

The discovery that the influenza virus mutates so rapidly explains why early vaccines were so ineffective. None of the vaccines created during the Spanish flu epidemic were of any use at all since they did not contain the flu virus. However, even today's flu vaccines—the only way we have of preventing the flu—tend to vary in their effectiveness because it is difficult to predict which strain will be the most common in any given year.

Inoculation is the technique of artificially infecting a person with just enough of a disease to make him or her sick but not enough to kill the person. Once the person has recovered, he or she will then be immune to the disease.

The Chinese had used powdered smallpox scabs, blown up the nose of a patient with a tube, to inoculate people against smallpox for centuries. In the Middle East, the method used was to scratch the patient's arm with a quill that had been dipped in powdered scabs. The practice remained generally unknown in Europe, however, until the early 1700s when Lady Mary Wortley Montagu, wife of the British ambassador to Turkey and a smallpox survivor, had her own children inoculated. Because of her tireless efforts to promote the new treatment, and the assistance of Caroline, Princess of Wales, inoculation gradually became a common practice among those who could afford it. During the Revolutionary War, General George Washington had all his troops inoculated and experienced no major smallpox outbreaks during the war.

Inoculation, however, had some serious drawbacks. After inoculation, the patient would develop a mild case of the disease; but sometimes he or she died from it. And during the period of the illness, the patient was highly contagious. What was needed was a method to gain the resistance inoculation brought without the risks of contagion or death.

An English doctor, Edward Jenner, thought he might have a solution. Among dairy farmers it was said that people who caught cowpox, a smallpoxlike disease of cows that did not kill humans, could not catch smallpox. In 1796, Jenner was able to inoculate a boy with cowpox taken from a milkmaid. The boy did not become seriously ill and later was found to be immune to smallpox. Jenner had found the magic shield against smallpox infection. He called his technique "vaccination," from the Latin words meaning "taken from a cow." Jenner's discovery led to the eventual eradication of smallpox in 1977.

Later, researchers such as Louis Pasteur discovered how to make a weakened form of a deadly virus and use it to inoculate people, who would then be immune to the disease. Influenza vaccines usually contain weakened forms of several strains of the influenza virus, to give people resistance to as many forms of the disease as possible. Early versions of the vaccine occasionally made people mildly ill, but present-day vaccines have no such side effects. One continuing problem with influenza vaccines is that they must be made almost a year in advance; if a new strain of the flu emerges, or a strain that the vaccine does not protect against becomes common, the vaccine will offer no protection. Still, if you think you are at risk of being infected by influenza during the flu season (late fall to early spring), you should be vaccinated.

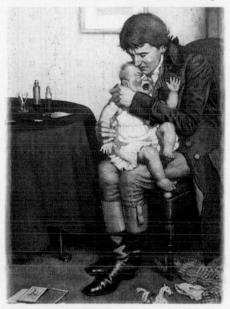

Edward Jenner administering an inoculation

Each year, scientists and doctors attempt to predict which flu strains will be common in the coming year and make vaccines that are able to fight those strains. However, since they must make the vaccines nine to ten months in advance, it is still possible that any of the strains will mutate into a type that the vaccine does not protect against. This is also the reason that, unlike other viral diseases like chicken pox or small-pox, a person who has caught the flu can still catch it a few years later; the virus has changed form and become one with which the body is not familiar.

The Spanish Flu: Renewed Interest

One question scientists still have not answered is why the Spanish flu was so deadly and killed people the flu does not usually kill. Instead of the flu's usual vic-tims—the very young and the very old—the Spanish flu killed young people in the prime of their lives. Why was this so?

One theory is that the immune response of the very young and elderly is different from that of adults and middle-aged people. Infants and young children tend to have a generalized response to infection that is weaker than that of adults. In adults, however, the immune system responds locally or directly to the area that is under attack and much more intensely than in older or younger people. The theory is that when confronted with a massive infection, the young adult body responds very strongly and the area becomes inflamed. When attacked by the Spanish flu, this intense local reaction was extremely dangerous because it caused the lungs to become very inflamed, filling up with too much blood and fluid. People actually drowned inside their own bodies.

Another theory is that the Spanish flu did not kill alone, but had a mutation that allowed it to work with a bacteria when it infected the host. Although this seems to be the mechanism of the swine flu that occurred after 1919, there is not enough evidence to prove this theory applies to humans. For one thing, sometimes there were no bacterial infections found in the people who were infected; for another, the experiments on ferrets in the 1930s did not show greater deadliness when a bacteria was introduced along with the flu.

Recently, expeditions have been mounted to regions of the earth that lie near the Arctic Circle in an attempt to retrieve specimens of the Spanish flu from bodies buried in ground that remains frozen all year long. It is hoped that a "live" virus (a virus that is still capable of infecting a living cell) will be found, so that study of the 1918–1919 strain can discover its peculiar deadliness.

One thing scientists do know is that the world is still not free of pandemic influenza. For many scientists, the question is not "Can another deadly influenza epidemic happen?" but "When?" They believe that by studying and understanding what made the Spanish flu so deadly, they may uncover clues that will help people fight very deadly influenza strains in the future.

THE POTENTIAL DANGERS OF INFECTIOUS DISEASE

Humans have always struggled against infectious diseases—diseases that can be spread from one person to another. For most of history, though, scientists have not understood how these diseases are spread. At first, people thought that the gods must be punishing people for doing something wrong. Often, people practiced ritual purity—special ways of cleaning themselves—to keep from becoming sick. Although we now know that people are not being punished by the gods when they get sick, this probably worked because keeping yourself clean is a good way to kill the germs that cause disease.

But regardless of the precautions that we have learned to use, throughout history there has continued to be one known disease that humans cannot seem to completely escape the ravages of: influenza. Understanding the mystery of influenza, which continues to haunt scientists, is vital not only to prevent its deadly return, but to understand how other plagues begin. Unfortunately, the outlook concerning our ability to understand and stop infectious diseases is rather bleak. In general, there appears to be a feeling of pessimism about eradicating any modern diseases—especially influenza because it mutates so rapidly.

The Illusion of Safety

Interestingly, for most of the twentieth century, people in the developed nations of the world thought of themselves as freed from the horrors of plague. Polio, which had once terrified millions, almost never occurs anymore. World War II was the first major war in history to be fought without the outbreak of an epidemic. Improved understanding of viruses and bacteria had created vaccines for many terrible diseases, such as tuberculosis. The discovery of antibiotics seemed likely to free humankind forever from pandemics. In 1977, thanks to a massive international effort, smallpox was eradicated from the world. Scientists talked about eradicating other diseases, like polio, in the near future.

So research essentially turned away from infectious disease and focused instead on heart disease and cancer, which had become the leading causes of death in most of the developed world. Infectious diseases just didn't seem like much of a concern for the modern world.

Infectious Diseases Are Back

But in the 1980s a new plague became a pandemic: AIDS. A disease that destroys the body's ability to fight off infection and has already killed millions throughout the world, AIDS is now seen as a worldwide crisis. And many scientists have recognized that it is very similar to influenza in its ability to mutate rapidly. It is believed that discoveries made about influenza may help uncover information about AIDS and vice versa.

But time has not been on our side. Although there have been many breakthroughs in the treatment of AIDS, a true cure, as well as a vaccine, still have not been discovered. Meanwhile, millions of

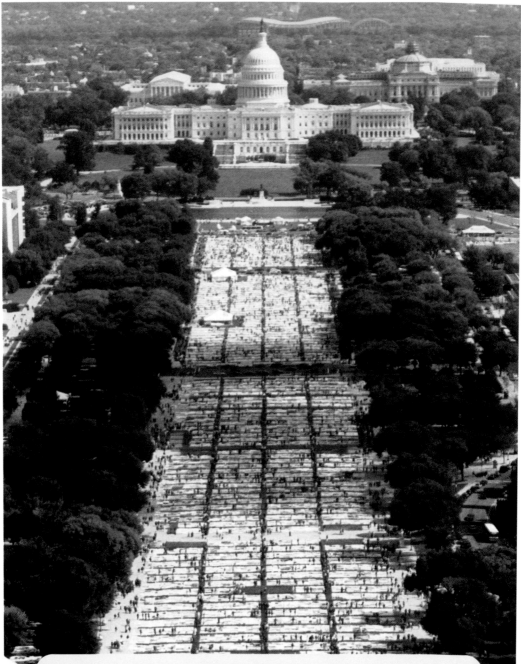

The AIDS Memorial Quilt, shown here stretched from the Washington Monument to the U.S. Capitol in 1996, was created in memory of those who have died of AIDS.

people worldwide suffer from the awful effects of AIDS and an emerging crop of new infectious diseases. Ebola, a highly contagious tropical disease that emerged in Africa, causes massive bleeding through the skin and internal organs, and has became famous for its swiftness and deadliness. Mysterious new diseases, such as the hantavirus that killed several people in the American West in the 1990s, have also been observed. And the unsettled conditions around the globe, with wars and internal conflicts raging in many portions of the world, have caused the widespread resurgence of many of the old plagues of humankind: cholera, typhus, and bubonic plague, to name a few.

More alarming has been the emergence of strains of diseases that are resistant to antibiotics. Tuberculosis, unseen for decades, made a frightening reappearance in many large cities, including New York, in the late 1990s. It is not impossible that influenza, or any other virus, could attack humans with the same sort of horrific results.

For all of these reasons, it is clear that people must continue to study the plagues of the past. As our understanding of diseases like influenza increases, we may be able to predict when a strain is likely to become incredibly lethal, and even how to treat it and create a truly effective vaccine. We must hope so and continue to learn more about the terrible autumn many years ago when a silent killer stalked the globe. We are learning the hard way that technology has not yet made us victorious in the war against epidemics.

GLOSSARY

alveoli   Tiny, delicate, air-filled sacs in the lungs where oxygen enters the bloodstream.

antibiotic   A drug that kills bacteria. Antibiotics have no effect on viruses.

antibodies   Special chemicals produced by the immune system to fight specific diseases.

bacteria   Microscopic parasites that infect living hosts and grow inside of them.

epidemic   An outbreak of a disease that infects many or most people in a certain area, such as a city or country.

host   The person or animal infected with a parasite.

immune system   The body's natural defense against diseases.

inoculation   Introducing a disease artificially into a person so that he or she becomes resistant to that disease.

pandemic   An outbreak of a disease that affects many people in a large region of the world.

pneumonia   Disease of the lungs and respiratory system, caused by a bacteria. Pneumonia can be fatal if not treated by antibiotics.

resistance   The ability of a person to keep from catching a disease. With many diseases, once a person has caught the disease, the person cannot catch it again.

staphylococcus   Bacteria that can infect the skin and mucous membranes.

streptococcus   Bacteria that can infect the respiratory system, causing a disease called strep throat. Strep throat is much more dangerous than a normal sore throat, and it can sometimes kill if it is not treated.

tissue   The groups of cells of a particular organ of the body.

vaccination   Inoculating a person with a weakened form of a disease so that the person will become resistant to the disease without either getting sick or infecting other people.

virus   A microscopic parasite, much smaller than bacteria. Viruses are not "alive" and can only reproduce within a living cell.

FOR MORE INFORMATION

In the United States

Centers for Disease Control and Prevention (CDC)
1600 Clifton Road
Atlanta, GA 30333
(404) 639–3311
(800) 311-3435
Web site: http://www.cdc.gov

World Health Organization (WHO)
Regional Office for the Americas
525 23rd Street NW
Washington, DC 20037
(202) 974–3000
Web site: http://www.who.int

In Canada

Clinical Trials Research Center
IWK Grace Health Center
5850 University Avenue
Halifax, NS B3J 369
(902) 428–8141
Web site: http://www.dal.ca/~ctrc

Health Canada
Laboratory Centre for Disease Control
Bureau of Infectious Diseases
Tunney's Pasture
AL 0913A
Ottawa, ON K1A 0K9
(613) 957-2991
Web site: http://www.hc-sc.gc.ca

Web Sites

Flu 101
http://www.flu101.com

Flu Watch
http://www.fluwatch.com

4Flu.com
http://4flu.4anything.com

National Foundation for Infectious Diseases
http://www.nfid.org

Pan American Health Organization
http://www.paho.org

FOR FURTHER READING

Aaseng, Nathan. *The Common Cold and the Flu.*
Danbury, CT: Franklin Watts, 1992.

Crosby, Alfred W. *America's Forgotten Pandemic:
The Influenza of 1918.* New York: Cambridge
University Press, 1990.

Farrell, Jeanette. *Invisible Enemies: Stories of
Infectious Disease.* New York: Farrar, Straus &
Giroux, Inc., 1998.

Foreman, Christopher H., Jr. *Plagues, Products,
and Politics: Emergent Public Health Hazards
and National Policymaking.* Washington, DC:
Brookings Institute Press, 1994.

Giblin, James Cross. *When Plague Strikes: The Black
Death, Smallpox, AIDS.* New York: Harper-
Collins, 1995.

Hays, J. N. *The Burdens of Disease: Epidemics and Human Response in Western History*. Piscataway, NJ: Rutgers University Press, 1998.

Iezzoni, Lynette. *Influenza 1918: The Worst Epidemic in American History*. New York: TV Books, 1998.

Karlen, Arno. *Man and Microbes: Diseases and Plagues in History and Modern Times*. New York: The Putnam Publishing Group, 1995.

Levinson, David, and Laura Gaccione. *Health and Illness: A Cross-Cultural Encyclopedia*. Santa Barbara, CA: ABC-CLIO, 1997.

McNeill, William H. *Plagues and Peoples*. New York: Anchor Books/Doubleday, 1998.

Watts, Sheldon. *Epidemics and History: Disease, Power and Imperialism*. New Haven, CT: Yale University Press, 1998.

INDEX

CREDITS

About the Author

Fred Ramen is a writer and computer programmer who lives in New York City. He is also the author of *Hermann Göring,* one of Rosen Publishing's Holocaust Biographies. Fred's interests include the American Civil War, science fiction, Aikido, and the New York Mets. He was a semifinalist in the 1997 *Jeopardy!* Tournament of Champions.

Photo Credits

Design and Layout

Evelyn Horovicz